YOUR KNOWLEDGE HAS VALUE

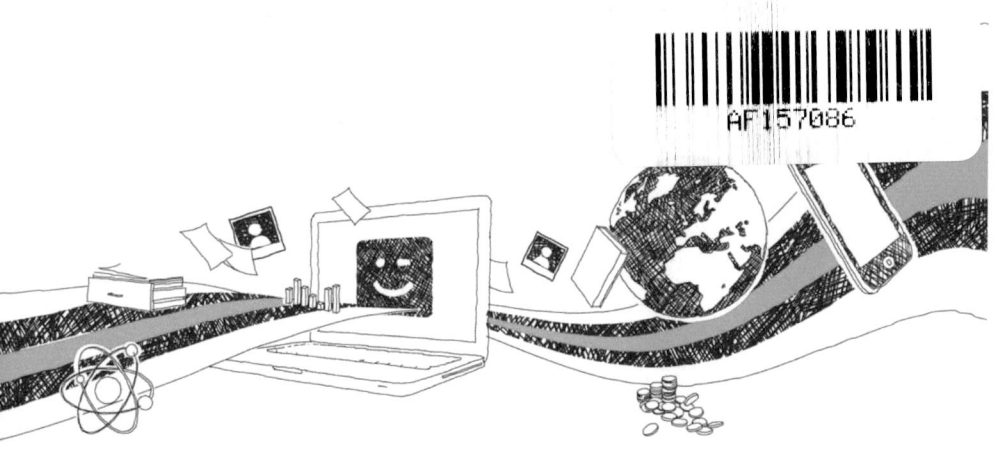
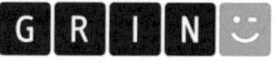

Carol Benjamin

Theory and Health Behavior Models and Theories

GRIN Publishing

Bibliographic information published by the German National Library:

The German National Library lists this publication in the National Bibliography; detailed bibliographic data are available on the Internet at http://dnb.dnb.de .

Imprint:

Copyright © 2010 GRIN Verlag GmbH
Print and binding: Books on Demand GmbH, Norderstedt Germany
ISBN: 978-3-656-55134-8

This book at GRIN:

http://www.grin.com/en/e-book/265463/theory-and-health-behavior-models-and-theories

GRIN - Your knowledge has value

Since its foundation in 1998, GRIN has specialized in publishing academic texts by students, college teachers and other academics as e-book and printed book. The website www.grin.com is an ideal platform for presenting term papers, final papers, scientific essays, dissertations and specialist books.

Visit us on the internet:

http://www.grin.com/

http://www.facebook.com/grincom

http://www.twitter.com/grin_com

Introduction to Theory and Health Behavior Models and Theories

Carol Benjamin

TUI University

Abstract

In this assignment I select an article from the Health Science literature that is written by Paul Ciechanowski and colleagues titled "Relationship Styles and Mortality in Patients with Diabetes". In this article data were collected and analyzed and I discussed whether the author discussed the theoretical framework upon which the research questions were formulated. I also answered whether the research questions were theory-based or instead derived from a specific problem statement. I also discussed if the researcher explicitly state assumptions that were drawn from the theoretical framework. To what extent was the methodology linked to a theoretical framework was also addressed. Finally, I discussed if the authors state whether their conclusions were consistent with existing theory and whether the authors discuss the development of new theory.

1. Did the author(s) discuss the theoretical framework upon which the research

   questions were formulated? Were the research questions theory-based? Or, were

   the research questions instead derived from a specific problem statement?

   Ciechanowski's and colleagues (2010) article discussed the theoretical

framework upon which the research questions were formulated. The article

reveals that prior research has shown that less social support is associated with

increased mortality in individuals with chronic illness. The authors set out to

determine whether lower propensity to seek support as indicated by relationship

style, based on attachment theory, is associated with mortality in patients with

diabetes. In this research the study is linked to a conceptual framework stating the

prior research that was already reported. Therefore this new study is linked to the

previous study. This study that the authors set out to complete has not yet been

explained scientifically so the authors choose to study this area of interest which

is built on the frame work that the pervious research was formed.

   A review of an article by Mitchell and Jolly (2007) shows that this

research question is theory-based. It is consistent with existing facts and it is

constructed by systematically collecting data and carefully analyzing the data for

patterns. From Mitchell and Jolly's article, this theory based research does not

ignore the facts and can make predictions that are counter-intuitive. This theory

can also suggest controversial, new ways of looking at the world.

   This article also helps in showing that this research question is theory

based since the theory summarize and organize a great deal of information and therefore has the ability to connect facts. This means that this research will not produce isolated bits of trivia. Instead the findings will fit into a framework that connects many other studies. The article by Mitchell and Jolly also shows that since theories are often broad in scope they can be applied to a wide range of situations and researchers can generate a wide variety of studies from a single theory. This research question is theory based since the theory can be tested and there are variables that can be objectively measured by making specific predictions.

2. Did the researcher explicitly state assumptions that were drawn from the theoretical framework?

   Ciechanowski et al. article explicitly state assumptions that were drawn from the theoretical framework. The article explains that attachment theory provides a theoretical, evidence-based model for understanding the propensity and ability of individuals to research out to others for support. This theory posits that all individuals develop a cognitive map based on prior experiences and determines ones comfort and ability to interact with or reach out to others, particularly at times of distress. The article explains that on the basis of empirical research in infants, children, and adults over the past 30 years, distinct relationship styles arising from these cognitive maps have been identified and demonstrate high levels of stability and continuity between early childhood and adulthood. The authors show that two of the styles, "dismissing" and "fearful" attachment style, are characterized by difficulty researching out for support or trusting others. Patients with these styles and characteristics have been described as having an independent relationship style. The authors explain that among

clinical populations with diabetes, 48 percent of patients are typically found to

have an independent relationship style while the remaining has an interactive

relationship style. These patients have greater comfort reaching out to others

although individuals with a preoccupied style are often characterized as being

highly dependent on others.

3. To what extent was the methodology linked to a theoretical framework?

The methodology that explains how the data was collected and how it was analyzed is

clearly linked to the theoretical framework to a great extent. The research shows a

collection of concepts from the previous research and this new research is built upon

it. The Group Health Cooperative which is demographically similar to the area

population was selected for the study. The original cohort for this longitudinal study

was sampled from adults who were at least 18 years from the Group Health

Corporative Registry who received care from one of the nine study clinics between

2000 and 2002. The diabetes registry database includes all Group Health Corporative

members meeting criteria such as filling prescription for insulin or an oral

hypoglycemic agents, two fasting glucose more than 126 mg/dl in 12 months, two

random plasma glucose level more than 200mg.dl, two outpatient diagnosis of

diabetes.

The relationship style was measured with participants completing the four-item

Relationship questionnaire and the participants were categorized as been

characterized by one of four attachment style. It is very clear that this new research

method is linked to the previous research. This methodology is chosen since the previous study shows less support is associated with increased mortality in individuals with chronic disease. The study is intended to prove that individual with diabetes which is a chronic illness have a lower propensity to seeks support as indicated by relationship style. As a result the method includes relationship style. This is associated with indication of less support that is associated with increased mortality. Previous research studied the mortality in individuals with chronic disease. In this new study the authors wanted to know another question that was not answered in the previous study.

In this study the authors wanted to know whether lower propensity to seek support as indicated by relationship style is associated with mortality in patients with diabetes. As a result the authors collected Washington States mortality data and used proportional hazards models to estimate relative risk of death for relationship style groups.

4. Did the authors explicitly state whether their conclusions were consistent with existing theory? Did the authors discuss the development of new theory?

Ciechanowski et. al did not state explicitly whether their conclusion is consistent with existing theory. However the authors' conclusions implied that the conclusion was consistent with the existing theory. In the authors' conclusions it revealed that a lower propensity to reach out to others is associated with higher mortality over five years. This is consistent with the existing theory that argues that less support is associated with increased mortality in individuals with chronic illnesses.

The authors argued that if they assume that the impact of independent relationship styles on poor outcomes could be significantly reduced using clinical strategies, then it is worth considering the public health benefits of such strategies. Therefore the authors suggested the development of new theories by stating that one way to explore such public health benefits is to get a better understanding of the adverse impact that an independent relationship style can have on a population of individuals with diabetes by comparing it to the impact of depression on health outcomes and mortality in patients with diabetes.

Reference

Ciechanowski, P., et al. (2010). Relationship Styles and Mortality in Patients with

Diabetes. <u>Diabetes Care</u>. 33(3) pg. 539.

Mitchell, M., Jolley, J. (2007). Advantage of using Theory to Generate Ideas.

Retrieved on July 18, 2010 from:

http://www.markwebtest.netfirms.com/Appendix/Theory_Appendix/Using_Theory.htm